Eyebrow Shapes: Styling Guide

How to Shape and Maintain Eyebrows

By: Dana Tebow

TABLE OF CONTENTS

Publishers Notes 3

Disclaimer 4

Dedication 5

Chapter 1- Discovering Which Eyebrow Shapes Fits You 6

Chapter 2- The Proper Way to Shape Eyebrows 9

Chapter 3- How to Shape Eyebrows without Plucking Them 12

Chapter 4- How to Shape Straight Eyebrows into An Alluring Arch 15

Chapter 5- How to Get the Perfect Eyebrow Shape Every Time 18

Chapter 6- Not Only Women Shape Their Eyebrows 21

Chapter 7- Easy Eyebrow Shaping Tips 24

Chapter 8- Are Eyebrow Shaping Classes a Must? 27

About the Author 30

Dana Tebow
PUBLISHERS NOTES

Speedy Publishing LLC

40 E. Main St., #1156

Newark, DE 19711

www.speedypublishing.co

Cover Artwork: 24 Hr. Designs Ltd.

Editing: Speedy Publishing LLC

Book design: Speedy Publishing LLC

ISBN:

This is a reprint book.

DISCLAIMER

This publication is intended to provide helpful and informative material. It is not intended to diagnose, treat, cure, or prevent any health problem or condition, nor is intended to replace the advice of a physician. No action should be taken solely on the contents of this book. Always consult your physician or qualified health-care professional on any matters regarding your health and before adopting any suggestions in this book or drawing inferences from it.

The author and publisher specifically disclaim all responsibility for any liability, loss or risk, personal or otherwise, which is incurred as a consequence, directly or indirectly, from the use or application of any contents of this book.

Any and all product names referenced within this book are the trademarks of their respective owners. None of these owners have sponsored, authorized, endorsed, or approved this book.

Always read all information provided by the manufacturers' product labels before using their products. The author and publisher are not responsible for claims made by manufacturers.

Dana Tebow

DEDICATION

This book is dedicated to my family.

CHAPTER 1- DISCOVERING WHICH EYEBROW SHAPES FITS YOU

Want to know what eyebrow shape suits you? More than likely it is the shape that your eyebrows already are. Not to sound cute, but most of us have eyebrows that may need some work but usually not major reshaping.

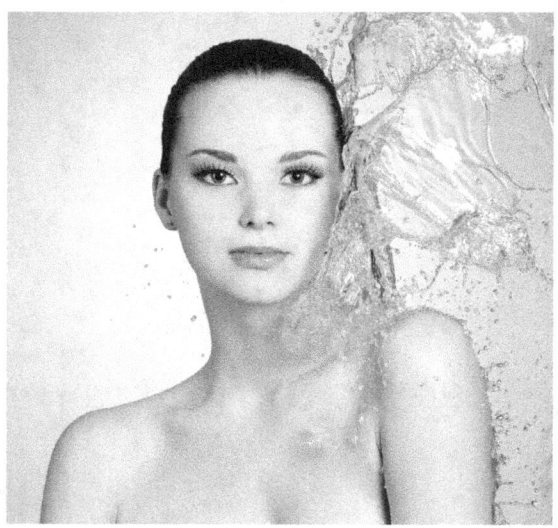

Hey you may love the way JLo, or Beyonce's eyebrows look, but that doesn't mean that the same shape, thickness and arch will look good on you.

So if you want to know what eyebrow shape suits you, you may want to start by looking in the mirror. Of course, if you aren't totally satisfied with your eyebrows there are many things you can do that don't require a total restructure.

Most of us can make dramatic improvement by simply adding a small amount of shaping and /or some thinning to our existing eyebrows. It can be a little more difficult to try to change the arch of your brows.

It's not impossible, of course, but if you have never done it before, it can be a challenge. And remember, if you mess it up you will look a little goofy until everything grows back.

To compound the goofiness you also have to remember that you will also need to even up both brows so they look at least close to the same shape, thickness and size.

So, if you want to do your brows yourself make sure that you allow enough time and I wouldn't recommend you try it for the first time right before a big occasion, just in case there is a problem.

So to get the best shape for you, you should probably just start with removing unwanted hair that is growing below, beside and above your main eyebrow line.

Just removing some extra "scruff" can make your eyebrows look more manicured and attractive. You may not even need to alter the shape or arch that much, you may just want to trim them so they are more defined and not so wild looking.

If you want to remove the unwanted hair for as long of a time as possible, you should either pluck or wax. You should not shave your eyebrows since this can actually promote more growth and you will just need to do more to keep your brows looking good... and who wants that?

Though plucking and waxing does hurt, it can also provide more of a permanent hair loss. Since you are taking the hair by the root, you won't have more hair growth until the hair can grow back from the root, and that will take upwards of two months.

Eyebrow Shapes: Styling Guide

Hey, you don't need to reinvent the wheel. More than likely your basic eyebrow shape is perfect for the shape of your face. You may just want to "neaten" your brows up a little bit to maximize how they look.

To find what eyebrow shape suits you just have a look in the mirror. If you want more than just a little "tidying up" you may want to find a professional to do it for you.

Chapter 2- The Proper Way to Shape Eyebrows

We know that we all have different facial shapes and features. One of the most easily changed, or enhanced, is the shape of your eyebrows. Your eyebrows have their own unique shape and arch and if you want to learn how to shape an eyebrow you can look no further than the nearest mirror.

Many people think that to learn how to shape an eyebrow also means they can completely reshape that eyebrow. In most cases you are much better off working with what you have.

This is about shaping, not re-shaping. Try to work within the natural shape of your eyebrows but just perfect it a little bit.

For example, many of us will notice some "scraggly" eyebrow hairs above, below or to the side of the main eyebrow. For the most part, this is what you want to get rid of. It's not about totally remaking the shape of your eyebrow but rather enhancing what you already have and removing any "overflow".

So, the first thing you need to do is have the proper tools handy. You can pluck your eyebrows with tweezers or you can use hot wax. Both methods work well, if you know what you are doing, it's really mostly just about preference.

Next, having a lighted and magnifying mirror handy will make the process easier. This will actually help in two ways: for one thing you will (obviously) be able to see better and for another, you can take a portable magnifying mirror anywhere in your home so you can work on your eyebrows in the room that has the best natural light.

Once you have your location and tools ready to go, look at yourself in the mirror. Concentrate on waxing your brows only to remove any excess hair above and below the main brow line. Don't try to reshape them; you are better off leaving that to a professional if that is what you want.

The same thing applies to plucking your eyebrows; concentrate on getting rid of any excess hairs but not so much on making changes to the overall line of the eyebrow.

If your eyebrow hair is overly long you may want to trim it. To do that, simply take a comb and run it through the eyebrow. Stop right at the end of the hair, while there is still some hair in the comb. Leave some hair that overhangs the edge of the comb and clip that off. Simple!

Sometimes we have eyebrows that are too thick, at least according to us. If that is your case you can also use the same method to make your eyebrows a little thinner. Just do the same steps but instead of waxing or plucking the "excess" hair above or below the main brow line, you can actually include a little bit of the main brow line.

One word of caution; if you get too carried away with one brow you will have to do the same thing on the other side. Make sure that when you are thinning your eyebrows you go very slowly and only take a small amount at a time.

Most of us are overly critical of our own appearance. Many times people think that there is something wrong with the shape or thickness of their eyebrows when the eyebrows actually fit very well into the overall shape of the face.

Dana Tebow

If you think that you must learn how to shape an eyebrow my advice would be to simply concentrate on shaping and not reshaping.

CHAPTER 3- HOW TO SHAPE EYEBROWS WITHOUT PLUCKING THEM

Many of us want an attractive manicured look but don't like dealing with the pain of plucking unwanted hairs. If you want to know how to shape eyebrows without plucking just keep reading.

If you want to know how to shape eyebrows without plucking you basically have two alternative methods; you can either wax your brows or use a fairly new technique called threading.

In this article I will explain a little bit about how each method works as well as the pros and cons of each so you can determine the best method for you:

1. Waxing is one of the methods that works well because the hair is actually removed from the root. That means it will be gone until the hair grows back. That process will often take up to two months.

Unlike shaving where the hair is only cut down to skin level, waxing, plucking and threading will actually pull the hair out by the root so you will have longer times between hair growth.

With waxing you can do it at home with a waxing kit or go to a hair salon or spa to have it done. The cost will depend on where you go. For the most part you will pay less at your hair salon than you would at a full service spa.

If you prefer to do it at home, you can do that too. You can go to any large store that sells cosmetics and buy a home waxing kit. You can usually heat the wax up in your microwave until it is the consistency of thick honey.

Dana Tebow

Once the wax is the right consistency you put in on the unwanted portion of hair on your brow. Then you apply a small piece of gauze to the wax.

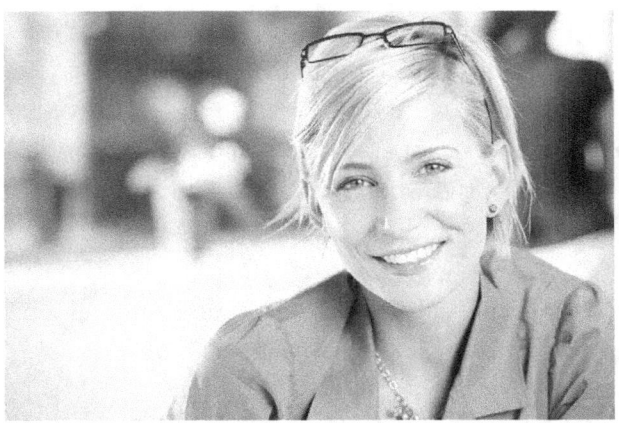

Once the wax has adhered to the gauze you quickly pull the gauze off in a fast, fluid motion. You pull in the opposite direction of hair growth.

And yes, this method does sting but unlike what you may see in the movies, it only stings for a few seconds and it's over with.

2. Threading may be fairly new to us, but it has been popular in some cultures for a long time. The basic concept is the same as waxing and plucking; you remove the unwanted hair from the root so it will stay gone for a few months.

The only difference is the technique you use to remove the hair. All you need is a piece of string that is at least 24 inches in length. It should be made of cotton and it should be strong so it does not break.

Tie the ends of the string together and double knot. Place your fingers in each loop of the thread. Turn the thread around itself several times until you see an "X" in the center of the thread where it crosses over.

Next, you will open the fingers of one hand while simultaneously closing the fingers on the other hand. The section of thread that is forming the "X" will move closer to the closed fingers.

After you've practiced this technique and are comfortable with it, you can than place the wound part of the thread directly over the unwanted hair.

When you start moving the thread by opening and closing your hands the thread will grab the hair and pull it out.

This method can be very effective, but out of all the methods, it is the one that will take some practice to get good at.

If you want to know how to shape eyebrows without plucking, this article should have shown you that you do have choices.

CHAPTER 4- HOW TO SHAPE STRAIGHT EYEBROWS INTO AN ALLURING ARCH

Our eyebrows are just one of those things about the way we look that is genetic. Some of us have perfectly shaped eyebrows, but most of us have eyebrows that we don't like. We think they are too thin, too thick or too straight. If you want to know how to shape straight eyebrows, keep reading.

Having a nice arch in your eyebrow tends to give your face more expression. It can also allow you more room for eye makeup. You can create very glamorous looks with eye makeup and having a higher brow and more eyelid to work with makes it that much easier.

But, some of you may be wondering how to shape straight eyebrows. If you were born with straight, thin eyebrows, keep reading for some tips on how to get that sexy arch you want.

One thing to keep in mind; this is not a process you want to rush through. If you make a mistake and wax or tweeze a big section of eyebrow you will need to do the same thing to the other side.

Yes, that will look weird, but it would look ever weirder if one eyebrow was significantly wider or thicker than the other. Go slow and concentrate on only one small area at a time for the optimum results.

Having a good magnifying mirror and a well lit room are also two important elements that will allow you to do a better job. Whether you decide you want to pluck with tweezers or wax with hot wax, have your supplies at hand before you start.

Here are the basic steps you want to follow:

1. First of all, make sure your eyebrows are clean and free of makeup or oils.

2. Then, brush your eyebrows. Brush them up towards your hair line by using either a lash brush or small toothed comb.

3. If you have any really long eyebrow hairs, use some scissors and trim them up. You don't want any "scragglies". It will also decrease the overall thickness of your brows which will make it less difficult to get the arched, sculpted look you want.

4. Take a pencil and place it along the bridge or your nose. Align the pencil so the top of it is aligned with your brow bone. Using a brow pencil, mark a small dot in the area where the top of the pencil is aligned with your brow bone. This should be the outer edge of your eyebrow.

5. Next, carefully take the pencil and lineup the end of the pencil with your nostril, angled toward the outer corner of your eye. This is where your eyebrow should end. Again, take a brow pencil and place a small dot in that exact spot.

6. Next, go to your mirror and look straight ahead. Line the pencil up with your eye so that your iris is directly behind the pencil. From that point you will gently roll the pencil outward, towards the outer corner of your eye.

Once the very inside edge of the pencil is aligned with the outer edge of your iris. Mark this spot on your eyebrow, it is where the arch should be.

Once you have the shape and you know exactly where your arch should be, you can start removing the hair and shaping the brow.

Dana Tebow

Now you know what to do and how to shape straight eyebrows, have fun!

CHAPTER 5- HOW TO GET THE PERFECT EYEBROW SHAPE EVERY TIME

There are a few things you can do to get perfect eyebrow shape for your face. Some of them will cost and some of them will be very cheap. It's up to you to decide how much you want to do yourself and what method you want to use.

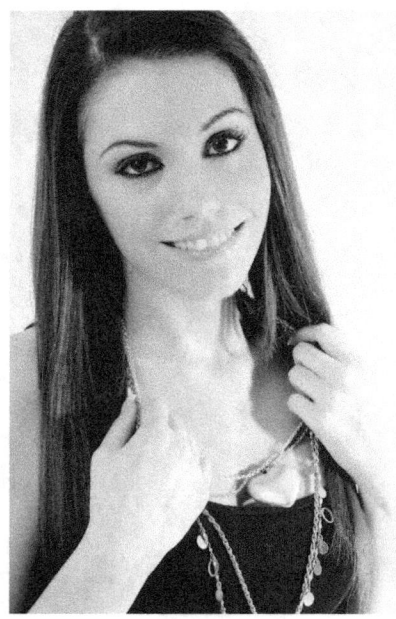

If you are willing to pay to have someone do it for you, you can most likely get perfect eyebrow shape for a small fee. How much the fee will be will be determined by where you live as well as the type of salon you go to.

For example if you go to a spa you will most likely pay a lot more for some eyebrow waxing than you would if you just had it done at the hair salon where you get your hair cut, colored or styled.

No matter where you decide to go, it may be worth it to have someone who has the right training and tools to do it for you. It can save you time and may make your eyebrows look even better than they do now.

Even so, if you want the job done right and done as quickly as possible you might be better off going to someplace where a professional could do it for you.

If you want to do it yourself your best bets are either plucking the unwanted hairs with tweezers or waxing them with a home waxing kit.

Both of these methods will produce long lasting results since you are actually removing the root of the hair. By doing it this way it will take about six to eight weeks to grow back. You don't have to mess with it all that often which is what most of us prefer.

To get it done right you should make sure that take a few things into consideration. For example, you want to make sure you have a lighted spot and a magnifying mirror.

Also, making sure that your face and eyebrows are clean and clear of oils will help. If you find that your eyebrows are too long in length you can easily take a sharp pair of scissors and trim off the length.

Don't go too crazy though, make sure you don't cut your eyebrows so short that they can't lay flat or you will look a little strange.

Once you get to this point, just examine your brows. Only start by taking off a little bit from spots that have excess hair. Don't take too much off too soon. Just start with those spots that are overgrown and kind of scraggly looking.

19

Remember, if you mess up you will have to live with it for at least a month or so. Be careful and take your time.

Don't mess up your eyebrows and have to hide inside your home for the next two months or so. Just make sure that when you start plucking or waxing concentrate on one small spot at a time.

And remember, to get perfect eyebrow shape you probably just need to clean up what you already have rather than completely change the shape, width and arch of your eyebrows.

CHAPTER 6- NOT ONLY WOMEN SHAPE THEIR EYEBROWS

Eyebrow shaping is not just for women anymore. More and more men are beginning to realize that the woman in their life likes the idea of a guy who isn't a slob. Many women prefer men who act like they care (at least a little bit) about the way they look. Gone are the days when women were the only ones expected to take time with their appearance.

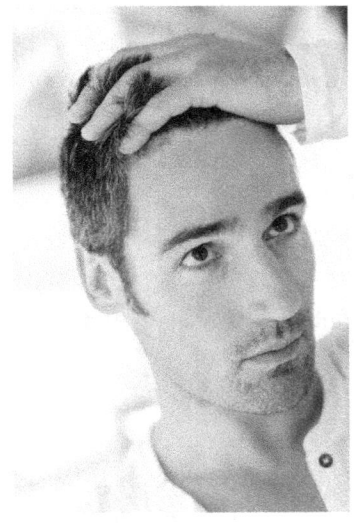

It doesn't matter if you are a man or a woman, there are some easy to follow tips for eyebrow shaping that will make it easier to get a great look:

1. First of all, if you can afford it, have a professional do it. In most salons you can get an eyebrow wax at the same time you are getting a haircut. The exact price will vary from one part of the country to another but for the most part, adding an eyebrow wax should be a fraction of the price of your haircut.

21

2. If you just can't afford to have it done for you, or if you are just one of those people who like doing things themselves, you can do it at home too. You can either use tweezers to pluck your eyebrows or you can use hot wax. Both methods work and each has it's own pros and cons so it is really just a matter of finding the method you feel most comfortable with.

3. Another tip you must keep in mind is that you should go very slowly while shaping your eyebrows. If you mess up and remove a big section of one of your eyebrows it will look twice as dumb because you will also need to make your other brow a similar shape and thickness (if you don't, it will look even worse!).

Make sure you go slow and work only with one very small section at a time to avoid waxing or tweezing off too much hair on your eyebrow.

4. Use a magnifying mirror and go to a well lit room in your home.

5. Make sure your eyebrows are clean and dry before you start.

6. Take some scissors and carefully clip any overly long hairs.

7. Next identify the basic shape of your brows. Most people should only try to remove excess hairs that are not part of the main brow rather than go crazy and try to totally reshape their eyebrows.

8. Slowly and carefully remove any excess hairs above or below the main brow.

9. And don't forget to target those hairs that are between your eyes so you aren't stuck with a uni-brow! Also, any stragglers to the sides of your eyes should be removed so you can end up with a fresh, neat eyebrow.

Dana Tebow

I've done it both ways; I have had my hairdresser do my eyebrow shaping for me and I have done it myself and I can tell you... she does a better job! If you can afford it, leave it to a professional. If you can't afford it, follow these tips.

CHAPTER 7- EASY EYEBROW SHAPING TIPS

No matter what method you use to remove unsightly excess hairs from your eyebrow line; plucking or tweezing, you will still need to get the shape correct. If you can find an eyebrow shaping diagram it will make the process more fool proof and easier.

If you can afford to have it professionally done, I would recommend it. They have the training and the tools to get the job done well. I'm not saying you can't or shouldn't do it yourself, I'm just a believer in making things as quick and easy as possible and having your eyebrows done by a professional seems like the best method.

In my experience, it doesn't cost much at all. I just have my hairdresser do it when I go in for a haircut. She only charges me a few dollars to do it. Some salons are pricier than others, I know, so it may cost you more, but ask to find out for sure.

If you want to do it yourself and you can find an eyebrow shaping diagram, it should go quicker and easier.

Everyone has their own unique shape to their face and eyebrows. For the most part, all you need to do is mimic the natural shape of your eyebrow and remove any unwanted hair that isn't part of the main brow.

You know, those unwanted hairs to the top, bottom or sides of your eyebrows. For most of us, just removing those on a regular basis is all that needs to be done.

Dana Tebow

At that point it is less about reshaping and more about trimming. You will also want to make sure that your eyebrows are clean, dry and free of makeup before you start.

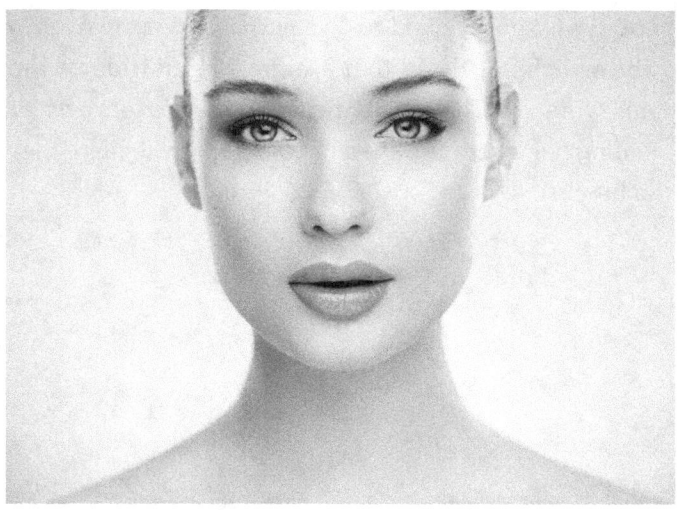

Also, if you opt to pluck your eyebrows rather than wax them, make sure you get quality tweezers. There really can be a difference between the qualities of tweezers.

A well lighted area of your home is going to provide the perfect location for the process. Also, having a magnifying mirror will make things easier too. These mirrors are often quite small and portable so you can take it to any place in your home. That makes finding the best light a much easier process.

If you have some hairs in your brow line that you don't want to remove but that are overly long, you can simply take a pair of scissors and cut it off a little bit. Keeping the length of all your brow hairs the same will give you a neater look too.

To determine if the length is OK simply comb your brows upward toward your hair line. Then you can easily snip off any overly long hairs before you begin waxing or tweezing.

Eyebrow Shapes: Styling Guide

Removing unwanted facial hairs and overly zealous eyebrows is one of those things that isn't hard to do but can really make a big impact on your overall appearance.

Most people will simply need to "clean up" and remove any overly long eyebrow hairs or those that are growing outside of the main brow line. Others will want to reshape their eyebrows and for them, finding an eyebrow shaping diagram will help make the process a lot easier.

CHAPTER 8- ARE EYEBROW SHAPING CLASSES A MUST?

There are several effective techniques you can use to trim and shape up eyebrows. Many of them will be learned while at cosmetology school or by taking some eyebrow shaping classes. As with most things, there is a bit of an art and a science to getting eyebrows that are the right shape.

Since everyone's face is a slightly different shape, to get the best overall look, the shape and arch of your eyebrows should be taken into consideration in the context of your face.

What do I mean by that? Simple, before you go running off in search of eyebrow shaping classes remember that you don't necessarily want your eyebrows to have the same arch and be the exact same thickness as a super model.

Your eyebrows probably already accentuate the shape of your face and you probably only need to make them a little neater by plucking or waxing any areas that are getting a little bit overgrown.

If you just have to make dramatic changes to your brows you may want to allow a professional the opportunity. After all, they have already been to class and they should know what they are doing.

Just to have a little eyebrow waxing or plucking done, it shouldn't be very expensive either. Many hairdressers can wax your eyebrows right before or after they cut and style your hair. Having it done in the same trip saves time and usually, money.

Most of the time, you will only pay a fraction of the amount you spent on getting your hair cut so you can probably afford to have a professional help spruce up your eyebrows.

If you do want to learn how to do it yourself there are many places you can go to learn. As I said above, if you want to make a career out of it, consider finding a cosmetology school in your area.

You may also be able to just take individual classes that only cover one thing, such as doing eyebrows, at your local community college.

You can always head online too. Again, if you just want to know how to do it but aren't really interested in making it your career you can probably just go online and look for videos, blogs or articles that will walk you through the process.

If you want to learn to sculpt your eyebrows yourself, here are some tips:

1. First of all make sure you remove your makeup and wash your face to rid your eyebrow area of all lotions, creams and oily substances.

2. Next get a good quality magnifying mirror and find a well lit spot in your home.

3. Take a small comb and comb your eyebrows up towards your hairline. If you see any really long eyebrow hairs just grab a sharp pair of scissors and carefully trim the hair to a little shorter length. Don't get too carried away, you don't want spiky eyebrows!

4. Slowly and carefully pluck or wax any overgrowth of hair. Any hair that is on the sides or top of the main line of your brow should be removed.

Dana Tebow

While this article was not the same as taking eyebrow shaping classes, it might give you a little help getting started.

ABOUT THE AUTHOR

Some women feel as though nothing looks good on them, and they never have anything to wear, THIS is not how Dana Tebow feels and elaborates more about this in her book. No matter your shape or weight, there are clothing styles that will work on your body. Spend some time evaluating your body. Be kind, gentle, and uncritical of yourself. This is not the time to get down about your belly or thighs. Simply take in what you have and learn how to dress it.

For instance, some women with broader, boyish frames feel they have a lot of trouble looking pretty and feminine. Many women with these body types suffer because most clothing for women is not cut to fit them in a flattering way. However, there are many fashion tips and tricks to achieve a style that is flattering and comfortable.

www.ingramcontent.com/pod-product-compliance
Lightning Source LLC
Chambersburg PA
CBHW061946280526
45787CB00004B/1746